ABOUT THE AUTHOR

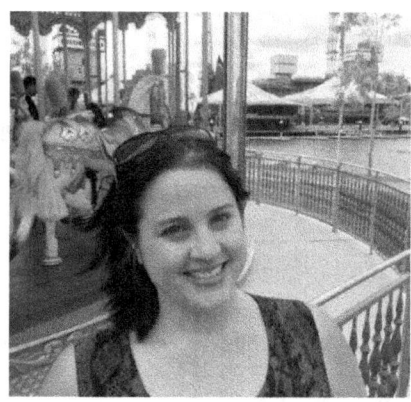

Thanks so much for purchasing "MSM Uncovered". My name is Jennifer Matthews and I am also known as Naturopath Jen. I am a qualified Naturopath, Law of Attraction Practitioner, Spiritual Life Coach and Self-Empowerment Educator. I have spent the last decade researching and spending thousands of dollars on my own personal development, as well as previously hosting multiple podcasts and blogs in the areas of health, wellness, mindset and spirituality.

I am now the founder and developer of the "Superconscious Success" Platform and the "Ask Naturopath Jen" Brand.

To learn more about myself and my journey (as it is quite an extensive read), please visit my personal site: http://www.spiritualcoachjenmatthews.com, where I delve into my purpose for writing these books and creating these brands and all the products/services (both free and paid) that can help you.

PREFACE

Are you suffering from constant pain and you have no idea how you are going to get some relief? Do you suffer with Osteoarthritis where the joint pain is crushing you? Are you suffering from hair loss or are you dealing with unhealthy, brittle hair? Do you have acne, wrinkles, cellulite or any other common skin condition? Are you looking for complementary therapies for cancer?

If so, then this book is for you. MSM may just be the answer you are looking for to help with all of the problems above, and much more...

ABOUT THE BOOK

MSM Uncovered is the second book in the ANJ Series because it is a supplement that I absolutely love and have a lot of faith in. With so many people suffering from a sulfur deficiency and not even knowing it, I thought it was definitely important information to get out there for those that are looking at optimizing their health.

This book will not only contain anecdotal information but will also have research articles spread throughout the book. They will not be in every section but will be in those where I could find some great research studies and where I think that section could do with clarifying.

OTHER BOOKS IN THIS SERIES

(All Available in Amazon under Naturopath Jen)

Magnificent Magnesium
Healing with Astaxanthin
Beginners Guide to Healing Leaky Gut Syndrome
The Acne Solution

DISCLAIMER

Please note that the information given in this book is for informational purposes only and is not intended to replace the advice of your health practitioner. If you experience symptoms that you are concerned with, please refer to your practitioner for further information...

****

SECTION 1 – INTRO TO MSM

****

Chapter #1 - MSM Basics

****

What is MSM?

MSM (Methyl Sulfonyl Methane) is a naturally occurring sulfur compound that is found in all vertebrates (including humans) and is highly effective in not only improving joint health and hair health but also in reducing pain relief significantly. It does this predominantly by reducing inflammation within the body.

How sulfur is absorbed into the diet is very interesting. MSM gets into the diet through the sulfur cycle. Plankton from the ocean will release sulfur compounds into the ozone and the ultra violet light will proceed to make MSM and its precursor DMSO.

These nutrients will then be returned to the earth's surface in the form of rain. When we eat the plants or the animals that have absorbed the MSM, the benefits begin to unfold.

Why Is MSM So Good for You?

- MSM is a potent antioxidant, anti-inflammatory and analgesic (pain reliever) which has been most known for its effect on joint health, pain management, hair health and skin health.
- As most conditions are caused from inflammation, MSM is highly effective at putting a stop to and/or helping to treat these common issues.

Signs of an MSM Deficiency

A deficiency in MSM has been shown to result in the following:

- Low Energy;
- Chronic Pain;
- Allergies;
- Low resistance to Stress;
- Parasites;
- Tissue and Organ Malfunction;
- Unhealthy Hair and Skin;
- Low Immunity.

A deficiency has also been shown to contribute to many conditions (see chapter 2 for further information on each of them), some of which include:

Asthma;
Arthritis;
Candida;
Diabetes; and
Constipation.

Nutritional Sources of MSM

As with any nutrient, it is always preferable to get it from naturally occurring food sources before taking supplementation. Unfortunately, this is not so easy when it comes to sulfur.
The foods richest in sulfur are those which we tend to not consume very much of in today's society, such as collagen or keratin.

However, Paleo is possibly one plan that would promote enough sulfur in the diet, as long as it is a paleo diet that emphasizes the quality of the foods as opposed to just the type of food.

Bone Broth

If you ever sat in the kitchen while your grandmother was making homemade chicken soup (as I did) or you remember your mum coming in with a nice pot of homemade chicken soup when you were sick (which I also did) then you would have been exposed to bone broth at some point in your life.

Bone broth is basically as the name implies. It is the boiling down of bones until all of the collagen and minerals seep into the water and then you drink it. It is absolutely delicious and so good for you.

One of the best sources of sulfur in our diet would be from the connective tissues in the bones of grass fed and free-range animals and therefore boiling down some bones into a bone broth and drinking the broth regularly could provide you with almost enough sulfur to promote optimal health.

The sulfur in the bones, and the amino acids proline/glycine are some of the components that make bone broth so great. So, to get you started with implementing MSM into your diet, how about I give you a bone broth recipe that you can get started using today…

Bone Broth Recipe

Ingredients:

1 kg or more of beef bones from grass fed cows;
2 chicken feet if possible (just gives that extra bit of gelatin);
1. onions;
2. carrots;
3 stalks of celery and any celery leaves you have;
2 tbsp. Apple Cider Vinegar;
1 tbsp. Celtic Sea Salt;
Any herbs of choice.

Methods:

1. Roast the beef bones in the oven for about 30 minutes at 200 degrees Celsius.
2. Place the bones in a large stock pot and pour filtered water over the bones and add the vinegar.
3. Let this solution sit for about 30 minutes or so as the acid from the vinegar will help to make the nutrients more available.
4. Roughly chop and add the vegetables to the pot and add any herbs and spices you are going to use.
5. Bring this broth to a boil. Once it has come to a vigorous boil bring it back down to a simmer. To simmer beef broth leave it for 48 hours and for chicken broth leave it for 24 hours.
6. Remove from the heat and allow it to cool slightly.
7. With a metal strainer, strain out all of the bones and vegetables.
8. When cool enough, store in a large glass jar in the fridge for up to 5 days or freeze until needed.

Raw Foods

MSM is in virtually all raw foods and is found in decent quantities in green leafy vegetables such as Brussel sprouts and kale. It is also found in garlic, onions and asparagus.

However, although vegetables can contain a significant amount of MSM, it should not be your primary source due to the poor amounts of sulfur in the soil that these vegetables are grown in.

Animal Sources

Eggs, Meat, Poultry, Fish and Milk are all a much more reliable source of MSM than Raw Foods.

Why Don't We Get Enough Sulfur in our Diets?

There are a couple of reasons for this. Firstly, as mentioned above, the richest source of sulfur is found in collagen and keratin and in modern society we seem to not consume too much of these.
However, thanks to more real food advocates they are becoming much better known, especially in the form of bone broths.

Secondly, MSM is lost significantly when the food is processed. Cooking, drying and steaming food depletes the MSM content, as does washing our food and storing it for a long period of time.

So, as you can see it is very difficult to get a sufficient quantity of MSM into your diet without a little additional supplementation, especially if you are wanting to receive therapeutic doses.

Supplemental Forms of MSM

MSM is able to be found in capsules, crystals, flakes, powders, tablets, lotions and gels. I prefer to use the crystals or flakes when I take it internally as it gets absorbed a lot quicker than tablets and capsules. I use lotions and gels when I require it to be absorbed through the skin (as is the case with muscle pains). If you would like to learn how to make your own lotions and gels, you can go to the recipes section at the back of the book.

Chapter #2 – Beneficial Supplements to Take With MSM

****

Vitamin C (Overall Health, Cell Regeneration)

The number one nutrient that has been shown to work extremely well alongside MSM is that of Vitamin C. In fact, by combining MSM and Vitamin C together, they work synergistically to provide the benefits listed in the upcoming chapters.

When MSM is taken alongside Vitamin C you will notice particular benefits:

1. Helps the body to build new cells.
2. Helps reduce scar tissue and wrinkles and helps keep the skin more elastic.
3. Helps the hair and nails grow stronger and faster.

Glutamine (Athletic Performance, Antioxidant Capabilities)

When used alongside MSM this nutrient is a great recovery workout combination. L-Glutamine is the most prevalent amino acid found in skeletal muscle tissue and blood and may significantly aid in muscle recuperation as well as overall immune function.

Just like MSM, Glutamine (when taken orally or intravenously) has been shown to raise the body's natural antioxidant glutathione.

Glucosamine (Arthritis and Joint Health)

When taken with MSM, this supplement has been shown to provide double the joint comfort relief than either of them alone. Previously you would find most arthritis supplements would contain Glucosamine and Chondroitin alone. However, since MSM has now been recognized as essential for joint health they have started adding that too.

Chapter #3 – Dosages and Toxicity
****

Optimal Intakes of MSM

As MSM is not stored in the body, a fresh supply is needed to prevent any further deficiencies developing. As you age your MSM concentrations also decrease so your requirement for it will be a lot higher.

It is important to start off slowly when taking MSM and gradually increase your dosage, so as to minimize any digestive complaints that might appear. So as to minimize the chance of heartburn, take MSM with your meals.

A single dose of MSM will not be a cure all but taken over time on a daily basis you will be able to start experiencing the amazing benefits of this nutrient.

A good way of increasing your supplementation is by incorporating the following tiers – although everybody is different, so you will just have to experiment yourself.

Tier #1
Start off by taking 500mg per day and take this dosage for a week.

Tier #2
Increase the dosage to 1000mg (1g) per day and take this dosage for a week.

Tier #3
Every day add on another 500mg per day until you reach 10000mg (10g).

Tier #4
Once you have been taking 10g per day for a couple of weeks and have made up for the years of deficiency then start to reduce it to a maintenance level.

Tier #5
For most people the maintenance level will be about 4-8g per day.

Note: *Make sure you drink plenty of water when starting on MSM and/or when increasing your dosage of MSM. Also ensure that you do not use tap water with the MSM as the chlorine in it can cancel the effectiveness of the MSM.*

Toxicity of MSM

MSM has been found to be safe with minimal reported adverse effects, even at very large doses. The only effects that have been reported (on minimal occasions) are loose stools, stomach upset or skin rashes, which could indicate a slight allergy to the product, but these symptoms will disappear once you have stopped taking the MSM.

In fact, there have been numerous studies done showing that MSM is Non-Toxic even at very large doses.

Research (1) – Non-Toxic for Pregnant Females even at extremely high amounts of 1000mg/kg/day (Animal Study)

Magnuson et al, *"Oral Developmental Toxicity Study of Methylsulfonylmethane (as OptiMSM®) in Rats."*, Food and Chemical Toxicology, 2006.

This study split the pregnant rats into 4 separate groups and were administered a variety of different dosages. There was no evidence of maternal toxicity and no significant differences in the litter viability, litter size or litter body weight upon testing. There were no foetal abnormalities seen in the MSM treated group or in any of the foetuses. Therefore, the non-observed adverse effect level for both maternal and developmental toxicity was 1000mg/day.

Please note that this study was done in rats and although the animal studies are generally very accurate and MSM is seen as extremely non -toxic for both the pregnant female and the foetus, it is still wise to either administer it at reasonably low doses (1-3g per day) and/or do it under the supervision of a practitioner.

Research (2) – MSM has very low toxicity (Animal Study)

Takiyama K et al, *"Single and 13 – Week Repeated Oral Dose Toxicity of Methylsulfonylmethane in Mice"*, Oyo Yakuri Pharmacometrics, 2010.

In this study they split the mice up into separate groups. One group was given a single dose of 2.5g per kg body weight, one group was given a single dose of 5.0g per kg body weight and the other group was given up to 10g/kg body weight over a period of 90 days. They found that with these numbers there was no toxic effects.

Detox Symptoms

When you first start taking MSM you may experience some detox symptoms which may make you want to stop taking it. But that could be a big mistake. The symptoms you experience can range from mild flu-like symptoms to more severe symptoms.

If the symptoms are not too severe try to tough it out for a few days and make sure you drink plenty of water. However, if you find the symptoms are too severe, try tiering the dosage down and take some hot baths to make you sweat more and therefore make the detoxification process go a lot quicker. Soaking in some Epsom salts is also a good idea.

More information on how MSM can help with detoxification can be found here...

People who should be cautious when taking MSM

MSM is extremely safe for most individuals and is actually about as toxic as water. However, if you have kidney issues or kidney disease it may be an idea to check with your practitioner prior to taking this supplementation.

Medications that are contraindicated with MSM

If you are taking high doses of aspirin or blood thinning medications such as heparin or dicumarol, it is advisable to check with your physician prior to taking MSM. This is because it has been observed in some clinical settings that it may have a blood thinning aspirin like effect on platelet aggregation.

Chapter #4 – General Benefits
****

This chapter is designed to give you some generalized benefits of MSM. For more detailed information on how MSM affects individual conditions and to read up on the research studies, you can find it in Chapter 3. But if you are preferring to just get an overview on what it is good for, then this chapter is for you…

Bone and Joint Care

MSM is a beneficial nutrient for joint health and has been researched most commonly on Osteoarthritis, although it is also effective for Rheumatoid Arthritis too. To read up more on this benefit, you can go to "Chapter 24 – Osteoarthritis".

Pain Relief

Apart from Joint Health, MSM is now most well-known for its effects on managing pain in a multitude of pain related conditions. To read up more on this benefit, you can go to "Chapter 25 – Pain Relief".

Blood Sugar Control

Due to sulfur being an important component of insulin, a lack of this vital nutrient can contribute to constantly elevated high blood sugar levels. To read up more on this benefit, you can go to "Chapter 14 – Diabetes".

Helps the Body Absorb More Nutrients

There are many nutrients that are unable to be absorbed unless they have a good supply of sulfur/MSM with it. Such vitamins include:

- Co-Enzyme Q10;
- Vitamin A;
- Vitamin D;
- Vitamin E;
- Pantothenic Acid;
- Selenium;

- Calcium;
- Amino Acids; and
- Enzymes.

Vitamin C is another one that suffers if MSM is not available. This vitamin does a lot of healing all by itself, but it requires sulfur otherwise it won't be able to toughen the capillary walls.

Increases Oxygen Availability to the Body

MSM is very effective at detoxifying and increasing the bloods circulation of oxygen and therefore helps to get oxygen into the blood a lot more efficiently with the same amount of work. This is great news for those that have difficulty breathing such as is the case with **Asthma** or for those with serious breathing conditions like **Emphysema**.

To read up more on this benefit, you can go to "Chapter 27 – Respiratory Health".

Improves Skin Health and Complexion

MSM is necessary for collagen production and is very effective at helping sagging skin, wrinkles and dry skin. It is also very useful at moisturizing cracked feet. It is especially beneficial when combined with Vitamin C.

To read up more on this benefit, you can go to "Chapter 28 – Skin Health".

Improves Flexibility

Research has shown that MSM is highly effective in improving joint flexibility, as well as skin and muscle tissue flexibility. By taking MSM you are also restoring the juiciness in the tissues.

Potent Detoxifier

MSM makes your cells more permeable, therefore allowing toxins and metabolic wastes to be easily moved out of the cells, and while at the same time allowing essential nutrients and hydration to move in. It also has a remarkable ability to break up the bad calcium due to the fact that it is a calcium phosphate dissolver.

To read up more on this benefit, you can go to "Chapter 13 – Detoxification".

Strengthens Hair and Nails

MSM provides the sulfur needed to produce collagen and keratin (both critical for the production of healthy hair and skin). It has also been shown to contribute to improved strength and thickness of hair and nails, which can be noticed in as little as two weeks of consistent use.

To read up more on this benefit, you can go to "Chapter 18 – Healthy Hair/Nails".

Natural Energy Booster

As mentioned previously, MSM increases the permeability of the cells. Because of this intestinal permeability, these cells require less energy to deal with all of toxins.

To read up more on this benefit, you can go to "Chapter 15 – Energy Improvement".

****

SECTION 2 – RESEARCH

****

Chapter #5 – Allergies

****

A damaging immune response by the body to a substance, especially foods, pollen, fur or dust, to which somebody becomes sensitive.

Types of Allergies

There are many different types of allergies that you may experience, including:

1.   Cat Allergies;
2.   Ragweed Allergies;
3.   Latex Allergies;
4.   Pollen Allergies;
5.   Shellfish Allergies;
6.   Peanut Allergies;
7.   Egg Allergies;
8.   MSG Allergies;
9.   Mosquito Bite Allergies;
10.   Dog Allergies.

How MSM Can Help with Allergies

MSM is known to not only aid in reducing inflammation within the body, but also in inhibiting histamine production.

Now don't get me wrong, MSM is not an anti-histamine. It inhibits the production by blocking the receptivity of histamine in the specific tissues associated with allergies, such as mucous membranes in the nasal passages. As histamine is responsible for causing the inflammation, swelling and fluid build-up that comes with allergies, taking MSM can alleviate those effects.

Also, when your body is deficient in MSM the cell walls can harden and hinder the fluid flow through the cell walls, therefore making it difficult for the foreign particles to flow out.

It may also be useful at reducing other symptoms associated with allergies, such as headaches, dizziness or chronic fatigue.

Environmental Allergies

If you find that you suffer not only from hay fever but also chemical sensitivities, dust mite allergens or pet allergies, then having MSM with you could be the key. In studies, subjects have found that although it may not completely eliminate allergic responses, it reduces the symptoms enough to be able to wean off of their anti-histamines.

Food and Drug Allergies

Studies have also shown that in individuals who have a tolerance to certain drugs such as aspirin, NSAID's, Anti- Arthritics and Oral Antibiotics, as well as those who have mild to severe allergies against various foods (gluten, cereals, shrimp, dairy etc) have a lessened intolerance or a complete tolerance to these foods after consuming as little as 1g per day over time.

Recommended form and dosage of MSM for Allergies

As stated above, people were able to reduce their need for allergy medications and reduce intolerance to certain foods purely by ingesting 1g of MSM per day. Therefore, ensuring that you ingest at least that 1g per day would be beneficial to alleviating allergies (more if possible).

Research (3) – Beneficial Effects of MSM on Seasonal Allergic Rhinitis

Barrager E et al, *"A Multi-Centered, Open Label Trial on the safety and efficacy of Methylsulfonylmethane in the Treatment of Seasonal Allergic Rhinitis"*, The Journal of Alternative and Complementary Medicine, 2004.

In this study 50 subjects consumed 2600mg of MSM orally per day for a total of thirty days. On days 7, 14, 21 and 30 their symptoms were evaluated. Plasma Immunoglobulin E and C - reactive protein were measured at baseline and on day 30, as well as another inflammatory marker, histamine.

As early as Day 7 showed significant improvements in upper respiratory and total respiratory symptoms, while lower respiratory symptoms were significantly improved by 21 days. These respiratory improvements continued throughout the 30 days. Energy levels also increased significantly by Day 14.

Chapter #6 – Antioxidant/Glutathione Production

****

A substance that reduces damage due to oxygen, such as that which is caused by free radicals.

MSM has been known to be a potent antioxidant, however it is now known that most of MSM's antioxidant actions are not because of the MSM itself but because of the effect the sulfur has on the production of the internal antioxidant "glutathione".

What is Glutathione?

Glutathione is a protein that is found inside every cell of the human body, especially that of the liver. It is known as a sulphuric tripeptide and it consists of the amino acid's glutamic acid, l-cysteine and l-glycine. Although it has been found that supplementing with glutathione itself is not readily absorbed, supplementing with l-cysteine, l-glycine or other sulfur compounds such as MSM is beneficial in increasing Glutathione levels within the body.

What are the Benefits of Glutathione?

Powerful Antioxidant

Being Glutathione's main claim to fame, its antioxidant capabilities are what makes it such a remarkable protein in the body.

Cancer Treatment

The antioxidant capability of Glutathione has been found to reduce the growth of cancer cells and Lipomas. Some doctors even recommend supplementation of Glutathione (through sulfur, Cysteine etc.) to treat cancer, as it increases the effectiveness of chemotherapy drugs and it also reduces their toxicity. To read more about how MSM helps cancer, go to "Cancer".

Detoxification of Heavy Metals

It has a remarkable ability to detoxify heavy metals from the body. To read more about how MSM helps detoxification, go to "Detoxification".

Infertility in Males

Glutathione is able to positively influence the quality of sperm in men, by decreasing the oxidative stress on the sensitive sperm and therefore minimizing damage to their DNA. It is therefore recommended that men trying to conceive take a supplement of Acetyl-L-Cysteine, and now even MSM so as to increase the production of Glutathione.

How MSM Can Help with Glutathione Production

sulfur is needed for the manufacturing of both Alpha Lipoic Acid and Vitamin B1, which are both important glutathione co-factors. MSM itself has been shown to up-regulate the activity of the glutathione enzymes in the presence of oxidative stress, such as is found after an intense exercise session.

Recommended form and dosage of MSM for Glutathione Production

How much MSM you take for Glutathione production would depend on what condition you are needing to heal. However, a minimum dosage I would recommend for optimal glutathione production would be 3g per day.

Research (4) – MSM Increases Liver Glutathione Levels

DiSilvestro R et al, *"Methylsulfonylmethane (MSM) Intake in Mice Produces Elevated Liver Glutathione and Partially Protects Against Carbon Tetrachloride-Induced Liver Injury"*, FASEB, 2008.

In this study they set out to determine whether an oral intake of MSM would affect the tissue levels of the internal glutathione, as well as resistance to chemically induced oxidative stress. They found that administering the MSM for 5 weeks produced a significant increase in liver glutathione levels (by up to 78%). However, a similar response was not seen in the kidney glutathione levels. They also showed that MSM was able to partially inhibit liver injury from toxic carbon tetrachloride (see section on Liver Disease.)

Chapter #7 – Anxiety/Depression

****

Anxiety – A feeling of worry, nervousness, or unease about something with an uncertain outcome.

Depression – A common mental disorder characterized by sadness, loss of interest or pleasure, feelings of guilt or low self-worth, disturbed sleep or appetite, feelings of tiredness and poor concentration.

How MSM Can Help with Anxiety/Depression

Many people have reported benefits from using MSM for Anxiety and Depression and have often seen results within hours and not days. MSM helps the body to deal with both physical and psychological stress and so is especially beneficial with treating psychosomatic disorders.

MSM has been reported to repair nerve damage which means less jitteriness in everyday life with less anxiety. Studies have also found that Depression can be partially attributed to sulfur deficiency.

Recommended form and dosage of MSM for Anxiety and Depression

The recommended amount of MSM to treat anxiety and depression will differ depending on the person. I would start off with 1g x twice per day and then increase it until you notice a difference.

Chapter #8 – Athletic Performance and Exercise Recovery

****

How MSM Can Help with Athletic Performance

There are many roles MSM can play in helping athletes perform at his or her best, recover from injuries a lot quicker and therefore allow them to get back to doing what you love the most.

MSM works on collagen and affects muscles and joints. It works directly on the cell itself and makes the cell walls more permeable therefore releasing toxins and absorbing nutrients more easily.

Pain Relief from Injuries

Injury is certainly a common part of an athlete's life, whether they are professional or amateur. Most sports injuries involve pain, redness, heat and swelling and after soft tissue injuries and micro tears, MSM will provide a source of bio available sulfur to support the tissue repair and regeneration. It also speeds up the relief from inflammation and promotes much longer lasting healing.

Tissue Regeneration and Recovery

In order for connective tissue to be healthy it requires a significant amount of sulfur. As athletes you place a lot of pressure on the joints, tendons, cartilage and other connective tissue, therefore causing significant wear and tear. The Organic sulfur from MSM can assist in the healing process and provide powerful musculoskeletal and respiratory support.
Increase in Energy

Many athletes report increased energy when taking MSM, due to its ability to support the metabolic processes within the body.

Recommended form and dosage of MSM for Athletic Performance and Recovery

There are a couple of ways that I would recommend you take MSM for Athletes. Firstly, you can take it internally of at least 3g per day and/or use one of the recipes in this book to create a cream that you can rub onto sore muscles/joints…

Research (5) – Beneficial effects of MSM on lowering exercise induced oxidative stress

Nakhostin-Roohi B, *"Effect of Single Dose administration of methylsulfonylmethane on oxidative stress following acute exhaustive exercise"*, Iranian Journal of Pharmaceutical Research, 2013.

In this study they set out to determine if a single dose supplementation of MSM attenuated post exercise oxidative stress in healthy untrained men. 16 untrained young men were placed into 2 groups – 8 in the MSM group and 8 in placebo.100mg/kg of body weight was given to participants prior to running on a treadmill for 45 minutes at 75% VO2 max.

3 markers of Oxidative Stress - Protein Carbonyl (PC), Uric Acid and Bilirubin were all decreased in the MSM group and the Total Antioxidant Capacity (TAC) was increased in this group.

This study implies that giving a single dose administration (100mg/kg body weight) is effective at lowering oxidative stress, but a long-term use could work even more effectively by also affecting GSH levels.

Research (6) – Beneficial effects of MSM on markers of exercise recovery and performance in healthy men

Kalman DS et al, *"Influence of methylsulfonylmethane on markers of exercise recovery and performance in healthy men: a pilot study"*, Journal of International Society of Sports Nutrition, 2012.

In this study, eight healthy men who are moderately exercise trained (exercising less than 150 minutes per week) were randomly assigned to ingest either MSM at either 1.5g per day for 30 days or 3g per day for 30 days (28 days before and 2 days after the exercise session).

Before and after the MSM intervention the subjects induced muscle damage by performing 18 sets of knee extension exercises. Markers such as muscle soreness, fatigue, blood antioxidant status and homocysteine (marker of inflammation) levels were measured using a variety of tests and protocols. The group taking 3g per day had the greatest reduction in soreness and only this group had increased total antioxidant capacity. Both groups had decreased homocysteine levels. This may be a good reason to consider integrating at least 3g per day into your daily dosages.

Chapter #9 – Autoimmunity

****

An Autoimmune Disorder occurs when the body's immune system attacks and destroys healthy body tissues by mistake.

Types of Autoimmune Disorders

There are many different types of autoimmune disorders. Some affect individual organs within the body, while others affect the whole body systemically.

Common Localized Autoimmune Disorders

- Addison 's disease (Adrenals);
- Autoimmune Hepatitis (Liver);
- Coeliac Disease, Crohn's Disease and Ulcerative Colitis (GI Tract);
- Diabetes Mellitus – Type 1 (Pancreas);
- Hashimoto's Thyroiditis or Grave's Disease (Thyroid);
- Multiple Sclerosis (Nervous System); and
- Myasthenia Gravis (Nerves and Muscles).

Common Systemic Autoimmune Disorders

- Rheumatic Fever;
- Rheumatoid Arthritis;
- Scleroderma;
- Sjogren's Syndrome;
- Systemic Lupus Erythematosus
- Kawasaki Syndrome.

Causes of Autoimmune Disorders

Although autoimmune diseases can be genetic in nature, they need a trigger to be able to manifest. This means that unless you have something trigger the autoimmune gene you may never get it, even if you are susceptible.

Common triggers of autoimmune diseases are:

- Nutritional Deficiencies;
- Environmental Pollution;
- Toxins;
- Mercury Toxicity;
- Fluoride Contamination;
- Stress; and
- Trauma.

On top of this it is found that people who have an autoimmune disease are often deficient in glutathione. Because you cannot take glutathione orally as is (as it will be broken down by the intestines), you need to take its precursors, MSM or Cysteine.

How MSM Can Help with Autoimmunity

MSM has been found to be very effective at fighting the inflammation arising from autoimmune reactions, where the body's immune system turns on itself.

Although there are two main autoimmune diseases which tend to respond very well to MSM (Scleroderma and SLE), it has also been found to be helpful in treating Chronic Fatigue, Primary Fibromyalgia Syndrome, Multiple Sclerosis and Rheumatoid Arthritis.

There are a couple of reasons that MSM is effective at helping with the healing of autoimmune diseases:

REASON #1

MSM increases the production of glutathione in the body which is often deficient in people with autoimmune diseases.

REASON #2

MSM can help with the elimination of multiple food allergies and insensitivities and therefore it can also help with reducing the burden on the body's immune system.

Autoimmune Diseases that respond very well to MSM

Scleroderma

This is a relatively rare autoimmune disease that affects the blood vessels and connective tissue. It is characterized by fibrous degeneration of the connective tissue of the lungs, skin and internal organs (i.e. kidneys and oesophagus).

Jacob – Medical Director for the Scleroderma International Foundation, found that MSM is able to ease the symptoms associated with this condition by normalizing collagen formation.

SLE (Systemic Lupus Erythematosus)

This is a chronic inflammatory condition that affects many systems in the body and it is characterized by vasculitis, renal involvement and lesions of the skin and nervous system.

Jacob also states that MSM is helpful at alleviating the symptoms of SLE.

Recommended form and dosage of MSM for Autoimmune Disease

The most effective form of MSM to take for Autoimmune Disease is the crystallized form (as with Antioxidants) at a dosage of a minimum of 3g per day and upwards and just increase until you notice improvement with it.

Research (7) - Beneficial Effects of MSM on Autoimmune Lymphoproliferative Disease

Morton JI, *"Effects of oral dimethyl sulfoxide and dimethyl sulfone on murine autoimmune lymphoproliferative disease"*, Proceedings of the Society for Experimental Biology and Medicine, 1984.

In this study mice that were prone to Autoimmune Lymphoproliferative Disease were given a diet which included 3% MSM as drinking water, from the age of 1 month. They found that the average life span of the control group (without MSM) was 5.5 months while the average life span of the MSM group was more than 10 months of age. This study suggests that MSM can provide protection against the development of autoimmune disease as it showed decreased anti-nuclear antibody responses, as well as a significant diminution of splenomegaly, lymphadenopathy and anaemia development.

Chapter #10 – Cancer

****

A disease caused by an uncontrolled division of abnormal cells in a part of the body, leading to malignancy in different tissues or organs.

How MSM Can Help with Cancer

MSM is gaining increasing interest in the subject of cancer and multiple studies have been done showing how beneficial it can be (see below). MSM has the ability to change a cancer cell into a non-malignant cell and therefore slow the rate of growth of cancerous tumors.

Cellular Matrix Study

The cellular matrix study (sulfur study) done in 1999 was inspired by a fatal type of breast cancer that has been reported to respond to organic sulfur. In this study they had their participants go to the store and purchase some MSM supplements.

However, their results were far from amazing. In fact, apart from some gastrointestinal distress there were no noticeable changes at all. What they found was that the supplements they were getting actually contained a multitude of additives which were interfering with the bio-availability of this amazing nutrient. So, in order for this supplement to work it must be in its purest form without any additional additives.

The Cellular Matrix Study had some amazing results when it came to cancer. By giving their participants 30g of sulfur alongside their chemotherapy had no side effects whatsoever. That means no nausea, no hair loss and no diarrhea.

They also found there was a reduction in cancer cell counts (reported by their oncologists). Lymphomas in particular have been found to respond exceptionally well to sulfur, both by decreasing pain and by decreasing the size of the tumours.

Webster Kehr from the Independent Cancer Research Foundation has stated that the "MSM/Vitamin C Protocol for Cancer" is synergistic with chemotherapy and therefore will make chemotherapy more effective and less damaging. However, he does specify that it is critically important that you get

Pure Organic sulfur and not a form of MSM that contains fillers and additives. If you go to my store I have sourced some great MSM for you that is pure…

According to Mr Kehr, MSM by itself is an excellent cancer treatment for advanced cancer patients as it has the ability to get rid of lactic acid in the bloodstream, kill microbes in the bloodstream and much more. However, when combined with vitamin C (as explained in chapter 1 of this book) it makes it even better as it turns it into a protocol that also has the ability to revert cancer cells into normal cells.

MSM is known to open the ports of the Cancer Cells for the Vitamin C to enter in and kill the dangerous microbes. Therefore, Vitamin C should be taken ½ hour after MSM.

To learn more about this protocol, you can go to: http://www.cancertutor.com/faq_msm/

Recommended form and dosage of MSM for Cancer

If you are suffering with cancer and you are currently going through a chemotherapy regime it is recommended to orally take 30g of Organic sulfur or Pure MSM per day (as per the sulfur study). Also, if you are treating malignant melanoma it may be worthwhile using the gel from the recipe section of this book and placing it on your melanoma a couple of times a day, and place a band aid over it so that the MSM can really penetrate deep.

Research (8) – Beneficial effects of MSM on Liver Cancer

Kim JH et al, *"Methylsulfonylmethane suppresses hepatic tumor development through activation of apoptosis"*, World Journal of Hepatology, 2014.

> This study was done to investigate the effects of MSM on Liver Cancer. This study was a mouse study that showed that Liver Tumor development was greatly inhibited in those treated with MSM, compared to those without it. Liver injury was also shown to be attenuated in those taking the MSM and the study suggests that MSM has anti-cancer effects by inducing apoptosis in liver cancer.

Research (9) – Beneficial effects of MSM with Breast Cancer

Lim EJ et al, *"Methylsulfonylmethane suppresses breast cancer growth by down-regulating STAT3 and STAT5b pathways"*, PLoS One, 2012.

This study was an animal study designed to investigate the mechanisms whereby MSM inhibits breast cancer growth in mice. By administering MSM to these mice over 30 days they found that there was a decreased expression of 4 major molecules involved in tumor development, tumor progression and metastasis (STAT3, STAT5b, IGF-1R, and VEGF). Therefore, the authors of this study conclude that a human trial should be done to determine if it is beneficial for breast cancer victims and as it is a non-toxic drug it can safely and ethically be undertaken as a human trial.

Research (9) – Beneficial Effects of MSM on Gastrointestinal Cancer (In Vitro)

Lim EJ et al, *"Methylsulfonylmethane suppresses breast cancer growth by down-regulating STAT3 and STAT5b pathways"*, PLoS One, 2012.

This study was conducted to determine cytotoxic effects of MSM on gastrointestinal cancer cell lines. Three different types of cancer cell lines – Human Gastric Carcinoma, Human Hepatocellular Carcinoma and Human Esophageal Squamous Cell Carcinoma were all treated with MSM and incubated for 24,48 and 72 hours. Testing was then done, and cytotoxicity was observed. What they found was that MSM had a cytotoxic effect on cancer cell lines, with Hepatocellular Carcinoma showing the greatest improvement. This study suggested that MSM may induce a cytotoxic effect on GI cancer cell lines by inducing apoptosis (cell death) and cell cycle arrest.

Research (10) – Beneficial Effects of MSM on Metastatic Melanoma (Animal)

Caron JM et al, *"Methyl sulfone induces loss of metastatic properties and re-emergence of normal phenotypes in a metastatic cloudman S-91 (M3) murine melanoma cell line"*, PLoS One, 2010.

This study was set out to determine whether MSM/Methyl Sulfone was effective at treating Metastatic Malignant Melanoma. In this study they took Cloudman S-91 mouse cells, as these cells are highly aggressive and metastatic, and they represent one of the deadliest forms of cancer. What they found in this animal study was promising. They found that malignant melanoma cells that were exposed to MSM demonstrated the loss of malignant cell characteristics and instead started to see characteristics of healthy melanocytes. Therefore, MSM may have clinical potential as a non-toxic agent effective against metastatic melanoma.

Chapter #11 – Candida Albicans

****

A Yeast like Parasitic Fungus that can sometimes cause thrush or can become systemic and cause a whole host of issues.

Candida Yeast Infection is an extremely common problem in the western world today and unfortunately is not recognized completely by the medical establishment.

Candida is a condition which, if not treated and eliminated completely can cause a whole host of issues.

Often when your body is over-run with candida you will have an allergy or sensitivity to the yeast and this will produce a number of medically unexplained symptoms.

Symptoms of Candida Albican's Overgrowth

1. Fatigue;
2. Irritability and Mood Swings;
3. Anxiety and Depression;
4. Unexpected Weight Gain;
5. Muscle and Joint Pain;
6. Excessive cravings for sugar;
7. Dizziness;
8. Diarrhea or Constipation;
9. Abdominal Bloating;
10. Difficulty Concentrating;
11. Earaches;
12. Breathlessness and Wheezing;
13. Frequent Coughs and Colds;
14. Multiple Skin Conditions like Acne and Eczema;
15. Headaches;
16. Rectal Itching; and
17. Much More…

Cause of Candida Albican's Overgrowth

Over-consumption of Sugar and Diabetes

The modern diet contains a lot of carbohydrates, which gives the yeast the sugar it requires to feed itself. This includes sugar itself, foods containing sugar and anything that may convert to sugar. A diet rich in sugar will depress your immune system leaving you vulnerable to this yeast. Moulds and yeast containing foods must also be avoided.

As Diabetes is also composed of elevated blood sugar levels people with Diabetes tend to suffer more frequently from yeast infections.

Overuse of Antibiotics

Although the antibiotics can kill the bad bacteria in the gut, they also kill off any beneficial bacteria you may have there. This can leave your body defenceless to harmful bacteria and fungi, including the yeast Candida. If you do need to take antibiotics, make sure you also take probiotics after the treatment to replenish the bacteria in the gut.

Excessive Stress

There are two ways that stress can affect the growth of Candida. Firstly, stress increases the level of cortisol in your blood which also raises your blood sugar. Candida will feast on this excess sugar and your weakened immune system will be unable to stop it. Secondly, excessive and prolonged stress can weaken your adrenal glands which are also an important part of your immune system. Weakened adrenal glands will cause you to drink cup after cup of coffee, putting you at even more risk of the Candida taking over.

Use of the Pregnancy Pill

Hormonal imbalances caused by the pill can cause an imbalance of the chemical required for the healthy bacteria to thrive. By taking the pill it opens the door for the candida to outgrow the beneficial bacteria. On top of that, the main component of the pill "Estrogen" is known to promote the growth of this yeast. This is the reason why women tend to get more yeast infections when on the pill.

Mercury in your Fillings

The mercury will leak from your fillings into your bloodstream and this has been shown to kill the beneficial bacteria in your gut, allowing Candida to take over.

Chlorine and Fluoride

Both Chlorine and Fluoride kill the beneficial bacteria in the gut, so it is important to try to avoid both of these toxic compounds wherever possible.

Supplements that can help with Candida

Although I don't necessarily recommend a lot of supplements, there are some that could help you with the elimination of Candida:

1. Molybdenum – Good for clearing the toxins;
2. Zinc – Boosts immunity;
3. Chromium – Deficiency can lead to sugar cravings;
4. Vitamin C – Boosts immunity, Repairs Tissue Damage and Assists MSM;
5. Vitamin B – Repairs nerves and adrenal stress.

How MSM can help with Candida

MSM is recommended as a cleanser as it normalizes the pH level of the blood, causing a more alkaline environment and making it very difficult for the bacteria and yeasts to thrive. It also prevents the roots of the candida yeast culture from penetrating the intestinal wall, therefore reducing the severity of the overgrowth.

Recommended form and dosage of MSM for Candida

Anecdotal reports have indicated that they take 2g of MSM per day to help with the Candida, so I would recommend starting with 2g of crystallized MSM per day as a minimum and work upwards if need be.

Chapter #12 – Constipation

****

A condition causing a difficulty emptying the bowels and is usually associated with hardening of the stools.

If you are suffering from constipation you will know how debilitating it can be and you may have tried everything you can think of to fix it, without much success mind you. Being unable to defecate can become very painful and in some cases can even lead to bowel obstruction, which is a very dangerous condition.

Causes of Constipation

1.   Changes in diet, exercise or lifestyle habits;
2.   Ignoring the urge to pass bowel movements;
3.   Being under enormous stress;
4.   Eating a low fibre diet;
5.   Not drinking enough fluids;
6.   Taking calcium or iron supplements;
7.   Taking medications containing codeine;
8.   Taking diuretics;
9.   Taking medications for depression;
10.   Taking some antacids.

Although very few studies have been done showing the beneficial effects of MSM and Constipation, there have been numerous reports that MSM has brought prompt relief for chronic constipation.

How MSM can help Constipation

One way that MSM may help with constipation is because of its interaction with the B Vitamins. MSM works with B Vitamins (particularly Thiamine – B1) to improve the muscle tone of your stomach and intestines. This will help to move food along more efficiently, which can then be seen by a patient's improvement with constipation after taking MSM.

Recommended form and dosage of MSM for Constipation

Although some have reported results in taking as little as 500mg per day of MSM, along with 1g of Ascorbic Acid, the sulfur study has recommended at least 1 heaped teaspoon (6g) per day. Therefore, I would recommend at least 3g per day and work upwards until you notice relief.

Chapter #13 – Detoxification

****

The process of removing toxic substances from the system so as to promote healing and optimal wellness.

Symptoms indicating you may require a Detox

There are numerous symptoms you may experience which could indicate you would benefit from a gentle detox:

Lymphatic System

- Frequent colds and flu's;
- Tiredness;
- Dark Circles under the Eyes;
- Cellulite.

Liver

- Bloating;
- Nausea;
- Indigestion;
- Furry tongue.

Lungs

- Congestion;
- Runny Nose;
- Constant Sneezing;
- Clogged Sinuses.

Benefits of Detoxification

Detoxification is beneficial if you are just wanting to optimize your health and it is recommended that everybody does a detox at some point. Unfortunately, our society is full of chemicals, toxins and additives that we are becoming exposed to and not even aware of every single day.

However, it is especially beneficial for those that are suffering from chronic conditions such as:

- Allergies;
- Asthma;
- Anxiety;
- Arthritis;
- Autoimmune Conditions;
- Chronic Infections;
- Depression;
- Diabetes;
- Headaches;
- Heart Disease;
- High Cholesterol;
- Low Blood Sugar Levels;
- Digestive Disorders;
- Mental Illness; and of course
- Obesity.

Although fasting has been used as a detoxification method for years, adding MSM into the plan at the same time can have remarkable benefits.

How MSM can help Detoxification

By making your cells more permeable, MSM allows toxins and metabolic waste products to be shuffled out of the cells, whilst still allowing essential nutrients and hydration to be moved into the cells.

When starting to take MSM as part of a detoxification protocol you may experience negative detoxification symptoms in the first 1-10 days whilst toxins are being flushed from the system. These could include diarrhea, rash and possibly even headache and fatigue. The worse these symptoms are the more toxic your body is and therefore the more MSM your body needs.

MSM is not only great as part of a mercury detoxification process, but also for the detoxification of pharmaceuticals from your system.

Recommended form and dosage of MSM for Detoxification

For detoxification purposes it is good to internally consume at least 3000mg twice per day, but you may need to work up to that starting with a lower dose of 750mg twice per day.

Research (11) – Beneficial Effects of MSM on reducing Acetaminophen Induced Toxicity.

Bohlooli S et al, *"Effect of methylsulfonylmethane pre-treatment on acetaminophen induced hepatotoxicity in rats",* Iranian Journal of Basic Medical Sciences, 2013.

In this rat study they set out to determine if MSM was helpful in reducing liver injury associated with excessive Acetaminophen usage. Prior to taking the drug, the rats received 7 days of MSM (100mg/kg body weight) and then on day 7 they were given an intraperitoneal injection of Acetaminophen. They then took blood 24 hours later to determine their level of liver injury. They found that the high dose Acetaminophen increased the liver injury but supplementing with MSM 7 days prior attenuated those effects.

Therefore, the findings of this study suggest that pre -treating with MSM prior to taking the acetaminophen could alleviate hepatic tissue injury (possibly through its sulfur and antioxidant effects). Taking MSM regularly could alleviate the effects associated with pharmaceutical drugs.

Chapter #14 – Diabetes

****

A disorder of metabolism causing excessive thirst and the production of large amounts of urine.

What is Diabetes?

Diabetes is a long-term condition that causes high blood sugar levels. In Type 1 Diabetes the body does not produce insulin. In Type 2 Diabetes the body does not produce enough insulin for proper function. T1 Diabetics need to take insulin while T2 Diabetics are able to reverse it by managing blood glucose levels.

Symptoms of Diabetes

- Frequent trips to the bathroom;
- Unquenchable thirst;
- Losing weight without trying;
- Weakness and Fatigue;
- Tingling or Numbness in your hands, legs or feet;
- Blurred Vision;
- Dry, Itchy Skin;
- Frequent infections;
- Cuts and bruises.

How MSM helps Diabetes

Sulfur is a requirement for the production of insulin and therefore carbohydrates will not be able to be converted into energy, therefore causing excess blood sugars in the bloodstream.

When the pancreas works too hard and fast to produce and carry insulin it can become injured and stop working correctly. The cells in the body then become rigid and non-permeable and the blood sugars that are not being absorbed into the cells saturate the bloodstream and create a high level of blood sugars. Taking MSM regularly assists the cells to absorb better and therefore allows the pancreas the opportunity to regulate better.

Recommended form and dosage of MSM for Diabetes

MSM taken at 10g per day can help to restore normal blood sugar levels to the cells.

Chapter #15 – Energy Improvement (Reduce CFS and Fibromyalgia)

****

Chronic Fatigue Syndrome – A debilitating and complex disorder that is characterized by profound fatigue that is not improved by bed rest and which may be worsened by physical and mental activity.

Fibromyalgia – A condition characterized by widespread pain and a heightened and painful response to pressure. Fibromyalgia almost always accompanies CFS.

When we talk about improvement of energy we are talking about the electron transport system and the mitochondria, as well as the two main conditions affected by energy deficiency (chronic fatigue syndrome and fibromyalgia).

How MSM helps with Energy

Electron Transport System and ATP

sulfur plays a role in the electron transport system, which are the energy factories of the cell and ultimately the body.

Decrease in Energy Requirement

Due to the fact that MSM increases the permeability of the cells and allows essential nutrients into the cells, less energy is required to deal with the accumulation of toxins.

This will result in more energy being directed towards activity and necessary healing. MSM will increase the absorption of nutrients so that the energy expenditure on digestion (takes up 70-80% of your energy every day) is also greatly reduced.

Reduction in Lactic Acid

Chronic Fatigue is caused by restricted aerobic metabolism, therefore increasing the anaerobic metabolism and producing more lactic acid in the muscles, leading to the pains associated with Fibromyalgia.

Often people with Chronic Fatigue will get a sudden burst of energy and so will use that energy to do something only to find that they are restricted and in pain for the next few days afterwards as the body has had to revert to anaerobic metabolism, and therefore excess lactic acid. MSM is an important nutrient when it comes to flushing the lactic acid from your system. By taking more MSM the toxins that cause soreness are flushed out of your body.

Oxygen Transport

When we discuss Chronic Fatigue Syndrome and Fibromyalgia one of the contributing factors include insufficient oxygen transport into the cells. However, by supplementing other molecules that can also transfer oxygen to the cells such as MSM.

Recommended form and dosage of MSM for Chronic Fatigue Syndrome and Fibromyalgia

Depending on the severity of your fatigue and judging by the studies Stanley Jacob presents in his book you can use anywhere between 5 and 30g of MSM internally per day. It might be an idea to start with 5g per day and move upwards until you notice a difference.

Research (12) – Study #1

Stanley Jacob et al, 1999, "The Miracle of MSM: The Natural Solution for Pain".

In his book, Stanley Jacob presented 3 case histories where 5, 10 and 30g per day of MSM reduced or eliminated fatigue and pain in fibromyalgia and chronic fatigue syndrome.

Research (12) – Study #2

Stanley Jacob et al, 1999, "The Miracle of MSM: The Natural Solution for Pain".

In his book, Stanley Jacob also referenced another case study which showed that a competitive athlete mixed equal amounts of MSM and Vitamin C powder and drank it in the morning. This gave him an incredible rush of energy, and considerably more than either one alone.

Chapter #16 – Eye Health Improvement

****

Glaucoma – This is not just one disease but a group of eye conditions that result in optic nerve damage, possibly causing loss of vision. It is most often caused from abnormally high pressure in the eye.

Cataracts – The clouding of the normally clear lens of the eyes which makes it a little like looking through a fogged up window.

How MSM helps Eye Health

- Strengthens the eyes;
- Prevents glaucoma;
- Prevents cataracts;
- Keeps the eyes young;
- Dissolve mucus accumulation;
- Keeps your eyes moist;
- Corrects dryness;
- Relieves strain;
- Relieves red eye;
- Clears up pink eye;
- Clears up sties;
- Clears up eye infections.

MSM softens leathery eye membranes and allows nutrients to penetrate through the cell walls. It removes waste particle build-ups (cataracts) and inside eye pressure, as seen in the case of glaucoma. It also improves vision, muscle tone, damaged blood vessels, floaters and even red spots.

The eye is an open mucous membrane and therefore it is incredibly important to keep the area cleansed. An MSM solution is very soothing and strengthening for tired eyes.

In fact, instead of using saline solutions how about using MSM eye drops as they provide soothing, lasting relief with no burning or stinging.

Recommended form and dosage of MSM for Eye Health

For Eye Health you could take some MSM internally at a dose of 2g – 6g but I would also recommend you make yourself some MSM eye drops, found in the recipe section of this book.

Chapter #17 – GERD

****

GERD is a chronic symptom of mucosal damage caused by stomach acid coming up from the stomach into the oesophagus.

Gastroesophageal Reflux Disease is a digestive disorder that affects the lower Oesophageal sphincter. When this sphincter is weak or relaxes inappropriately, the stomach contents will flow back up into the oesophagus causing GERD.

Symptoms of GERD
- Heartburn (most common);
- Regurgitation (most common);
- Pain with swallowing/sore throat (less common);
- Increased salivation (less common);
- Nausea (less common);
- Chest pain (less common);
- Coughing (less common).

Causes of GERD
- Appearance of a Hiatal Hernia – Weakens the LES and causes GERD;
- Food Allergies – Especially in children;
- Hypercalcemia;
- Scleroderma and Systemic Sclerosis;
- Medicines such as prednisolone;
- Cigarette Smoking – Relaxes the LES;
- Obesity;
- Pregnancy; and
- Abnormal biologic or structural factors.

How MSM helps with GERD

Because of the ability of MSM to neutralize stomach acids, it can be a very effective treatment for Indigestion and GERD.

Recommended form and dosage of MSM for GERD

MSM is a nutritional supplement that has been shown to be effective in stabilizing the digestive process by ingesting 3g per day minimum.

Chapter #18 – Hair and Nail Health

****

MSM has been touted as the "Beauty Mineral" that provides the essential collagen and keratin required to produce healthy hair and nails. It has been found to contribute towards exceptional strength and thickness of the hair and nails and this has been seen in as little as a couple of weeks of consistent use.

Basics of Hair Growth

Your hair grows in three separate cycles:

- Growing (Anagen);
- Resting (Catagen); and
- Shedding (Telogen).

Every single hair on your head and body is in one of these phases at all time. You may not notice significant shedding because you will find the other hairs on your body are in one of the other two phases at the same time.

How quickly your hair grows is genetically determined, unless you make one change... If your growing phase lasts two years and your hair normally grows ½ an inch per month, then your hair will only grow 12 inches in the whole growing phase. However, if your growing phase lasts three years, then your hair will grow 18 inches.

How MSM helps with Hair and Nail Growth

Now if you have issues with growing your hair and nails, MSM is a perfect answer. Because MSM helps with tissue repair, some sellers tout it to promote the growth of hair and nails. MSM also helps your body build collagen – the protein that keeps skin and hair supple.

Recommended form and dosage of MSM for Hair and Nail Growth

Not only are you able to take it internally but you can also find specific creams/shampoos for hair growth that contain the nutrient – OR you can make your own. Apart from increasing the length of your hairs growth phase by stimulating scalp circulation, it is also useful at providing the chemicals necessary for nourishing the hair follicles.

If you would like to know how to make your own hair growth shampoo incorporating MSM into it you can go to the recipes section...

It is suggested to take at least 1.5g of MSM per day orally and increase up to 5g per day. Combine the MSM with at least 500g of Vitamin C for even better results. Some people notice a reduction in hair shedding and an increase in hair growth very quickly while others may take a few months. Be patient and increase the dosage as you see fit.

Also, if you sign up for my mailing list at http://www.asknaturopathjen.com/innercircle, I will notify you as soon as my book on hair loss and hair health is out.

Research (13) – MSM on Hair and Nail Health

Ronald M Lawrence, MSM and Hair/Nail Health.

Unfortunately, at the time of printing there are not that many scientific studies out there about the effects of MSM on hair and nail health.

However, a doctor by the name Ronald M Lawrence performed a couple of double-blind placebo controlled pilot trials to identify how MSM affected hair and nail health.

Trial #1 – Beneficial Effects of MSM on Hair Health

This study consisted of 21 subjects, 5 women and 16 men and it showed that 100% of the subjects put on MSM showed increased hair growth compared to the group on placebo, compared to only one subject on the placebo that showed an increase in hair length.

30% of the subjects showed an improvement in hair shine and brilliance, whilst none on placebo did.

Nail Health – Beneficial Effects of MSM on Nail Health

This study consisted of 11 subjects, 10 women and 1 man and showed that 50% of the subjects on MSM showed an increase in nail length and nail thickness compared to the group on placebo (Only 10% Improvement). None of the subjects on placebo showed an increase in nail thickness.

These trials went for 6 weeks. If the trial was able to go for more like 16 weeks the results would have been even better.

Chapter #19 – Indigestion

****

Pain or discomfort in the stomach that is associated with a difficulty digesting foods. It is not a condition in and of itself but it is a collection of symptoms that appear after eating.

Symptoms of Indigestion

Symptoms will vary from person to person and the frequency of the symptoms will also differ. Some people will experience indigestion occasionally, whilst others will suffer from it daily.

- Early fullness during a meal;
- Uncomfortable fullness after a meal;
- Discomfort in the upper abdomen;
- Burning or Bloating in the upper abdomen; or
- Nausea.

Causes of Indigestion

- Overeating or eating too quickly;
- Consumption of fatty, greasy or spicy foods;
- Too much caffeine, alcohol, chocolate or carbonated beverages;
- Smoking;
- Anxiety; or
- Certain antibiotics.

Conditions causing Indigestion

- Gastritis;
- Peptic Ulcers;
- Celiac Disease;
- Gallstones;
- Constipation;
- Intestinal Blockages etc…

How MSM helps Indigestion

Because of the ability of MSM to neutralize stomach acids, it can be a very effective treatment for Indigestion and GERD.

Recommended form and dosage of MSM for Indigestion

MSM is a nutritional supplement that has been shown to be effective in stabilizing the digestive process by ingesting 3g per day minimum.

Chapter #20 – Irritable Bowel Syndrome

****

A widespread condition involving recurrent stomach pain and diarrhea/constipation and is often associated with stress, depression, anxiety or infection.

Symptoms of IBS

Irritable Bowel Syndrome is a common disorder which affects the large intestine and commonly causes symptoms such as:

- Cramping;
- Abdominal pain;
- Bloating;
- Gas;
- Diarrhea; and
- Constipation.

Causes of IBS

Although the cause of Irritable Bowel Syndrome is not known, there are a variety of factors that may play a role. The walls of the intestines are lined with layers of muscle which relax and contract in a co-ordinated rhythm upon eating foods.

However, sometimes this rhythm gets jumbled up and you end up with contractions that are stronger and last longer than normal, therefore causing gas, bloating and diarrhea. However, on the other end is when you get weak contractions slowing the passage of food and leading to chronic constipation.

Triggers of IBS

Foods

Food allergies and intolerances can play a part in IBS. Although it is not yet understood completely, there are many people that suffer more after eating certain foods. The foods that seem to cause the issues are chocolate, hot spices, fruits, beans, cruciferous vegetables, dairy, soft drinks and alcohol. If you have IBS it may be an idea to first do an elimination diet to figure out what is contributing.

Stress

During periods of extreme stress, you may find that your IBS flares up. Your symptoms may be worse or more frequent during periods of increased stress. Although stress aggravates the condition, it is not the cause of it.

I believe that stress was a major contributor towards the development of my IBS. I was preparing for a wedding, organizing a move to Germany and working long hours at my place of employment at the same time, on top of subjecting my body to excessive exercise. Once all of that was over and I had moved to Germany my IBS miraculously disappeared.

Hormones

Many women find that their symptoms of IBS are worse around their menstruation and as twice as many women seem to get IBS than men, it is likely hormones play a role.

Candida Overgrowth

A common cause or trigger of IBS is a Candida overgrowth. MSM is very effective at removing candida from the body…

How MSM helps IBS

As MSM reduces inflammation throughout the body, and in this case the large intestine, it seems to be effective at reducing symptoms associated with Irritable Bowel Syndrome.

Recommended form and dosage of MSM for IBS

To help relieve the symptoms associated with IBS, start off with a dose of 2g per day, split up into 2 separate doses and increase up to 10g as needed, until you notice significant improvements in symptoms.

Chapter #21 – Leaky Gut

****

Hyper permeable Intestines – Holes in the lining of the intestines…

Leaky Gut Syndrome is becoming more researched in recent times and has been linked as being one of the major contributors towards autoimmune conditions.

On top of that they have found that leaky gut may be contributing to allergies, asthma, arthritis, inflammation, skin problems, headaches, energy issues, slowed metabolism and much more.

So, what is Leaky Gut then?

In a healthy gut, our intestines will contain a lining that is impermeable and tight knit and will stop toxins, unhealthy bacteria, food particles and GMO's from leaving the intestines and entering the bloodstream.

However, when we suffer from Leaky Gut Syndrome holes begin to appear in this lining and therefore toxic substances enter the bloodstream and cause a whole host of issues, including inflammation…

Symptoms of Leaky Gut Syndrome

- Bloating;
- Gas;
- Cramping;
- Pain;
- Aches; and
- Food Sensitivities.

Causes of Leaky Gut Syndrome

Diet

A diet high in refined sugars, processed foods, preservatives, refined flours and additives introduces chemicals to the body that is seen as toxic. These toxins start to build up and cause inflammation.

Chronic Stress

Chronic Stress suppresses the immune system and causes the body to be overrun with pathogens. This will cause gut inflammation and therefore lead to increased permeability of the intestinal lining.

Medications

Certain medications irritate the intestinal lining and decrease the mucosal levels, which can start the inflammatory process. A major example of this would be the pain reliever Ibuprofen.

Yeasts

As soon as yeast begins to get out of hand it mutates into candida which begins to make its own holes in the lining.

Zinc Deficiency

A lack of zinc is crucial for maintaining a strong intestinal lining. Studies have shown that supplementing with zinc when deficient can improve intestinal lining integrity.

How MSM helps Leaky Gut Syndrome

MSM can be very helpful in the treatment of Leaky Gut Syndrome by coating the mucous membranes in the body and preventing allergens and toxins from entering the bloodstream.

Recommended form and dosage of MSM for Leaky Gut Syndrome

For Leaky Gut Syndrome I would suggest 6g of MSM per day, split up into 2 separate doses and increase it as needed.

Chapter #22 – Liver Disease

****

Liver Injury is a type of damage to or disease of the liver.

When talking about Liver Disease, you are either talking about Acute Liver Injury or Chronic Liver Injury.

Acute Liver Injury

Acute Liver Injury usually occurs as a result of toxic metals, medication use and a number of acute illnesses. As the liver is able to repair itself, with treatment (MSM is one of them) your body should be able to recover full function within 8-10 weeks. That is, as long as Chronic Liver Injury has not occurred.

Symptoms of Acute Liver Injury

- Nausea;
- Loss of Appetite;
- Fatigue;
- Diarrhea.
- Vomiting;
- Feeling Unwell.

Causes of Acute Liver Injury

- Acetaminophen Overdose;
- Prescription Medications;
- Herbal Supplements, such as kava, ephedra, skullcap and pennyroyal;
- Hepatitis, Epstein Barr Virus, Cytomegalovirus and Herpes Simplex;
- Toxins;
- Autoimmune Hepatitis;
- Rare metabolic diseases such as Wilson's Disease.

Chronic Liver Injury

Chronic Liver Injury on the other hand is a lot more serious and although it progresses over time, it can kill somebody very quickly. As it happens over time the symptoms are much less than with acute, as are the causes.

Symptoms of Chronic Liver Injury

- Jaundice;
- Bleeding Easily;
- Pain in your upper right abdomen;
- Abdominal Swelling;
- Disorientation/Confusion; and
- Sleepiness.

Causes of Chronic Liver Injury

- Hepatitis B;
- Hepatitis C;
- Long Term Alcohol Consumption;
- Cirrhosis (formation of scar tissue in the liver); and
- Liver Cancer.

How MSM Can Help Liver Disease

According to numerous studies, MSM is effective at protecting the liver from damage caused by prescription medications, excessive pain killers or other toxic chemicals.

There are a few different ways that MSM is able to protect against acute liver injury:

REASON #1

They have found that MSM raises the antioxidants produced within our own body, SOD and CAT, therefore protecting against different types of acute liver injury.

REASON #2

As MSM help to create new healthy cells and the liver is able to repair itself, MSM is able to speed up the healing process within the liver.

REASON #3

If you have a liver disease such as Cirrhosis or Hepatitis C, MSM will help to soften the tissue in the liver so as to help prevent further scar tissue formation and therefore prevent hardening of the liver.

Other Supplements Useful for Acute Liver Injury:

#1 - Milk Thistle

The Number One Recommended Herb for Liver Health

#2 – Artichoke

Shown to support the liver and gallbladder function through the removal of toxins and the maintenance of healthy bile function.

#3 – Turmeric

Helps to protect the liver from damaging free radicals and promote a healthy inflammatory response.

Recommended form and dosage of MSM for Liver Injury

If you are suffering from Liver Disease it is advisable to get yourself to a therapeutic dose of 10,000mg per day, split up into two 5g lots. Start off slow (as per "Dosages" section) and work up until you reach this amount. After a few weeks, reduce down to 4-6g per day. According to the sulfur Study one member even reported regenerating his liver in 15 months after suffering 25 years from hepatitis C. He took 2 tablespoons (24g) of MSM per day.

Research (14) – Beneficial Effects of MSM on acute liver and lung injury (Animal Study)

Amirshahrokhi K et al, "*Effect of methylsulfonylmethane on paraquat induced acute lung and liver injury in mice*", Inflammation, 2013.

In this mouse study they set out to determine the effect of MSM on acute liver and lung injury. A single dose of a toxin called PQ was given so as to induce this acute injury and then the mice were given 500mg/kg of MSM per day for 5 days. At the end of this time the mice were ethically euthanized and then the lung and liver tissues were gathered to determine the injury caused.

What they determined with this study was that MSM decreased the liver and lung damage caused by this toxin and increased beneficial markers such as SOD, CAT and GSH compared to the PQ group.

Research (15) – Beneficial Effects of MSM on acute liver injury (Animal Study)

In this study they set out to determine if MSM was going to be useful against carbon tetrachloride (toxin) induced livery injury. A single injection of this toxin induced an increase in ALT and AST (indicator of liver damage) and also decreased SOD and CAT (antioxidants) in the body. After this toxin was given to the rats they also found an increase in pro-inflammatory cytokines and a decrease in anti-inflammatory cytokines.

This study showed that MSM raised the effects of the antioxidants SOD and CAT and it possesses a hepato protective effect against carbon tetrachloride liver injury in the rats.

Chapter #23 – Oral Health

****

There are benefits of MSM in healing gum disease. According to Dr Stanley Jacob, MSM is effective at healing a variety of oral issues:

Painful Tooth Root Infection

Although tooth root infections are considered incurable and dangerous, Stanley demonstrates the infection healing potential of MSM through the story below…

Research (12) – MSM helps with Painful Tooth Root Infection

Stanley Jacob et al, 1999, "The Miracle of MSM: The Natural Solution for Pain".

In this story, an 80-year-old woman had 3 teeth root canalled 25 years earlier and developed a serious infection. This infection became so painful that it started keeping her up at night. Even after doing multiple rounds of antibiotics, the infection would come back as soon as the antibiotics wore off. So she started taking 12g of oral MSM per day, as well as applied MSM crystals to her gums twice a day.

The pain and inflammation lessened every day, allowing her to sleep a lot better and within 2 weeks her infection was much improved. Six months after starting the MSM all the pain was gone, and the infection was healed.

Gum Disease

Dr Stanley Jacob believes that MSM offers an additional weapon against gum disease. Taking a daily dose of MSM of 2-8g, as well as using an MSM mouth wash or rubbing MSM crystals onto the inflamed gum tissue has been shown to help patients suffering from Gingivitis and Pyorrhoea.

Miscellaneous

On top of the Infections and Gum Disease, MSM has been observed to be useful in whitening the teeth and reducing tooth sensitivity.

How MSM helps Oral Health

MSM reduces inflammation of the gums, therefore preventing gingivitis and periodontitis.

Recommended form and dosage of MSM for Oral Health

When it comes to Oral Health and treating infections and abscesses, try working your way up to 12g of oral MSM per day. On top of that it is recommended to create your own mouthwash by taking a teaspoon of MSM and 100mls of water and then gargle the MSM in the mouth for a few minutes prior to spitting it out. Try not to swallow as it could contain toxins from your mouth in it.

Chapter #24 – Osteoarthritis

****

Degeneration of joint cartilage and the underlying bone, causing pain and stiffness – especially in the hip, knee and thumb joints.

Symptoms of Osteoarthritis

- Pain – Joints may hurt during or after movement.
- Tenderness – Joints may feel tender when you apply pressure to it.
- Stiffness – Joint stiffness may be most noticeable upon waking up or after inactivity.
- Loss of Flexibility – You can't move your joint through a full range of motion.
- Grating Sensation – May hear or feel a grating sensation when you use the joint.
- Bone Spurs – These hard bumps may form around the affected joint.

Causes of Osteoarthritis

Osteoarthritis occurs when the cartilage which cushions the ends of the bones in your joints gradually deteriorates. If the cartilage wears down completely, you are left with bone rubbing on bone and causing extreme pain.

How MSM helps Osteoarthritis

Research has shown that MSM is highly effective in improving joint flexibility. Additionally, it helps to produce flexible skin and muscle tissue. This leads to an increase in overall flexibility due to a restoration of the "juiciness" in the tissues.

Osteoarthritis can lead to joint pain and swelling. Joints that are affected by Osteoarthritis suffer from uneven loading and causes cartilage to build up to compensate for the uneven load. This will cause roughening and deformities in the joint surface and it will cause the joints to inflame and no longer operate smoothly. The outgrowths of the cartilage and bone causes a friction which creates pain and inflammation.

MSM has been shown to lower pain in many conditions including osteoarthritis and other joint disorders.

Sulfur has been found to be critical to joint health and MSM is known to deliver sulfur to the body in a usable way.

Recommended form and dosage of MSM for Osteoarthritis

As shown by the research studies given below, people have been put on anywhere from 1.5g per day and up to 6g per day. Start off with the lower dose and then continue to increase the dose until the symptoms improve. Although some people achieve results in a very short period of time, others may take a little longer so be patient...

Research (16) – Benefit of MSM with Osteoarthritic Knee Pain

Kim LS et al, *"Efficacy of Methylsulfonylmethane (MSM) in Osteoarthritis pain of the knee: a pilot clinical trial"*, Osteoarthritis Cartilage, 2006.

Fifty men and women (40-76 years) who all had Osteoarthritis knee pain were split up into two groups. One group was given 6g MSM per day and the other was given a placebo for 12 weeks. In this study they found that there was a decrease in pain and an improvement in physical functioning, as well as an improvement in the ability to perform daily activities.

Research (17) – Benefit of combining MSM with Glucosamine for Osteoarthritis

Usha PR et al, *"Randomised, Double Blind, Parallel, Placebo Controlled study of oral glucosamine, methylsulfonylmethane and their combination in osteoarthritis"*, Clinical Drug Investigation, 2004.

This study consisted of four different groups, each consisting of approximately 30 patients. The groups were split up into MSM only, Glucosamine only, MSM and Glucosamine together and Placebo. They were each given 1500mg per day for a total of 12 weeks and at the beginning and end of this time the levels of pain and the levels of swelling were measured.

What they found in this study was that although MSM by itself and Glucosamine by itself produced a great decrease in pain of Osteoarthritis sufferers, combining the two resulted in an even greater decrease in pain.

Research (18) – Benefit of MSM with Degenerative Arthritis

Lawrence RM, *"Methylsulfonylmethane (M.S.M.) a double-blind study of use in degenerative arthritis"*, International Journal of Anti-Ageing Medicine, 1998.

In this study 16 patients suffering from degenerative arthritis were split into two groups and one group (8) was given 2250mg per day and the other (6) was given a placebo for an unspecified period of time. This study showed that there was a better than 80% control of pain within 6 weeks of beginning the study.

Chapter #25 – Pain Relief

****

MSM is a potent analgesic (pain relief) and anti-inflammatory supplement and it has been proven to provide pain relief for people who are unable to achieve it any other way.

Common conditions that MSM is known to treat include back pain, joint pain, headaches and fibromyalgia.

How MSM helps with Pain

MSM has a number of pain-relieving qualities:

Regeneration of Body's Tissues

Sulfur is vital to the creation and regeneration of the body's tissues. When rigid, fibrous tissue cells swell and become inflamed, pain will result from the pressure surrounding it. MSM is important for restoring this flexibility and permeability of the cell walls, allowing fluids to pass through the tissues with ease.

Anti-Inflammatory

It is also responsible for reducing systemic inflammation.

Blood Vessels

MSM has been shown to dilate blood vessels and enhance blood supply, therefore speeding up the arrival of nutrients involved in the repair of the damaged tissue.

Muscle Cramps and Spasms

MSM has been shown to lower muscle cramping and consistent muscle pain.

Recommended form and dosage of MSM for Pain Relief

According to the study below it is advised to consume anywhere between 5g and 30g to deal with intense pain, but that will all depend on what you are trying to treat.

Research (12) – MSM Helps Fibromyalgia and Chronic Fatigue Syndrome Pain

Stanley Jacob et al, 1999, "The Miracle of MSM: The Natural Solution for Pain".

In his book, Stanley Jacob presented 3 case histories where 5, 10 and 30g per day of MSM reduced or eliminated fatigue and pain in fibromyalgia and chronic fatigue syndrome.

Chapter #26 – Parasites

****

An organism that lives in or on a second organism (host) and usually causes harm.

Most anti parasitics out there are poisonous chemicals that are designed to kill parasites and can often come with serious side effects.

Symptoms to indicate you may have Parasites

- Lowered Immune System and constant illness;
- Constant Tiredness;
- Difficulty Sleeping and Waking Up;
- Bloating and Gas;
- Allergies;
- Food Sensitivities;
- Recurrent bladder infections;
- Intestinal Cramps;
- Muscle or Joint Aches and Pains;
- Constipation or diarrhea.

How MSM helps with Parasite Removal

MSM is a great supplement to use for eliminating intestinal parasites. However, unlike other anti-parasitics, it actually works by forming a slick lining along the walls of your intestines and stomach. This coating will then bind to receptor sites in the mucus membrane (where parasites attach). As the parasites no longer have a place to attach, they will simply fall off and be eliminated through the normal elimination process.

There are many different parasites that can be removed, including Giardia, Trichonomas, Roundworms, Nematodes, Enterobius and Other Intestinal Worms.

Recommended form and dosage of MSM for Parasite Removal

To remove parasites from your body it is advisable to take 2g x 2 times a day (4g per day).

Chapter #27 – Respiratory Health/Sinusitis

****

Sinusitis is an extremely painful condition that can be benefited with the use of MSM.

How MSM helps with Respiratory Health

MSM helps to strengthen the lungs and possibly regulate the fluid that covers the surface of the airways. It helps to improve the elasticity of the lung cells and the permeability of the membranes which allows more oxygen to pass through.

Research - MSM Benefits Emphysema and Lung Tumors

> In this study, 7 subjects with respiratory deficiencies were given MSM in amounts of 250 – 500mg per day. 5 of these subjects had emphysema and 2 had lung tumors. Both were on radiation and chemotherapy prior to including MSM in the diet but they were not receiving any benefits from it.
>
> Before and during the test period the subjects with emphysema were required to walk a distance that was within their physical capabilities. Within 4 weeks of starting their ingestion of MSM, these emphysema sufferers had doubled their comfortable walking distances.
>
> The subjects in the tumor group were assessed as being more alert and have a better attitude than before the test.

How MSM helps with Sinusitis

MSM is a powerful pain reliever and as such is a great solution to inflamed sinuses.

Recommended form and dosage of MSM for Respiratory Health and Sinusitis

If you are suffering from some respiratory ailments, start off with at least 1g per day and increase your dose until you notice improvements. If you are suffering from sinusitis, check out our Sinusitis remedy at the end of this book.

Research (3) – Beneficial Effects of MSM on Seasonal Allergic Rhinitis

Barrager E et al, "A Multi-Centered, Open Label Trial on the safety and efficacy of Methylsulfonylmethane in the Treatment of Seasonal Allergic Rhinitis", The Journal of Alternative and Complementary Medicine, 2004.

In this study 50 subjects consumed 2600mg of MSM orally per day for a total of thirty days. On days 7, 14, 21 and 30 their symptoms were evaluated. Plasma Immunoglobulin E and C - reactive protein were measured at baseline and on day 30, as well as another inflammatory marker, histamine.

As early as Day 7 showed significant improvements in upper respiratory and total respiratory symptoms, while lower respiratory symptoms were significantly improved by 21 days. These respiratory improvements continued throughout the 30 days. Energy levels also increased significantly by Day 14.

Research (14) – Beneficial Effects of MSM on acute liver and lung injury

Amirshahrokhi K et al, "Effect of methylsulfonylmethane on paraquat induced acute lung and liver injury in mice", Inflammation, 2013.

In this mouse study they set out to determine the effect of MSM on acute liver and lung injury. A single dose of a toxin called PQ was given so as to induce this acute injury and then the mice were given 500mg/kg of MSM per day for 5 days. At the end of this time the mice were ethically euthanized and then the lung and liver tissues were gathered to determine the injury caused.

What they determined with this study was that MSM decreased the liver and lung damage caused by this toxin and increased beneficial markers such as SOD, CAT and GSH compared to the PQ group.

Chapter #28 – Skin Health Improvement

****

MSM is necessary for collagen production and therefore is great for your skin. It works together with Vitamin C to build new, healthy tissues and it can normalize collagen formation, radically improving skin health.

How MSM helps the Skin

Reason #1 – Helps Dry Skin

MSM softens the skin, making it smoother, hydrated and much more flexible. Therefore, if you have chronically dry or mature skin that has lost most of its elasticity, then MSM is for you. It makes the cells more permeable and so is much more receptive to plumping and hydration. Taking MSM internally can also help with the cell permeability.

Reason #2 – Helps Inflammatory Skin Conditions

The sulfur compound also has an anti-inflammatory and skin-repairing effect, which may be useful for inflammatory skin conditions such as eczema, acne and psoriasis. It also may help smooth and soften acne scars and hasten the healing of existing lesions.

Reason #3 – Helps Diminish Hyper-pigmentation and Age Spots

MSM has been shown to reduce Hyper-pigmentation issues such as melisma, scarring, age spots, freckles and sun damage. This will work both when taken as an internal supplement and also as an external application. The best results have been achieved when used topically.

Reason #4 – Reduces Wrinkles

MSM actually helps to rebuild and maintain healthy collagen levels, which means fewer wrinkles and crows feet.

Recommended form and dosage of MSM for Respiratory Health and Sinusitis

In order to keep supple healthy skin, it is recommended to consume at least 1-3g per day, up to 6g per day for chronic skin conditions.

Chapter #29 – Snoring

****

To breathe during sleep with a rough, hoarse noise due to vibration of the soft palate.

Symptoms of Snoring

- Loud, harsh or hoarse noises;
- Waking up with a sore throat;
- Waking up with a dry throat.

Causes of Snoring

Sleep Apnoea

One of the most common causes of snoring include Sleep Apnoea. Some symptoms associated with sleep apnoea include:

- Excessive daytime sleepiness;
- Choking or gagging while you sleep;
- Pauses in breathing;
- Morning headaches;
- Difficulty concentrating;
- Moodiness, Irritability or Depression;
- Frequent need to urinate at night.

Obesity, Pregnancy and Genes

Extra tissue in the throat can vibrate as you breathe in air in your sleep, which can cause you to snore. People who are obese or pregnant can cause you to have extra bulky throat tissue. Genetic factors such as enlarged tonsils, large adenoids, long soft palate or long uvula.

Allergies, Congestion and Certain Nasal Structures

Anything which prevents you from being able to breathe properly through your nose can cause snoring. This can include congestion, allergies or deformities in the nasal septum.

Alcohol, Smoking, Aging, Drugs and Medications

Substances that cause your tongue or throat muscles to relax can cause you to snore.

How MSM helps with Snoring

Although the actual process is not well known for how MSM benefits snoring, apart from its potent anti-allergy effects on the upper respiratory system, there is a study showing that it may be beneficial.

Recommended form and dosage of MSM for Snoring

To reduce snoring start off by taking 2g of MSM Orally 1 hour before going to bed and titrate up as need be. It would also be an idea to use the nasal spray given in the recipe section about 15 minutes prior to sleep.

Research (19) – MSM and Snoring

Jacob S, "Pharmacologic Management of Snoring".

In this study they showed that 35 subjects who suffered from chronic snoring were given a 16% water solution administered in the form of a nasal spray 15 minutes before sleep. There was a significant reduction in symptoms in 80% of the subjects.

8 of the subjects that had relief from MSM had their MSM replaced with Saline and 7 of the 8 patients resumed snoring within 24 hours of taking it. After the MSM treatment was restored they all showed a significant reduction once again.

Chapter #30 – Stomach Ulcer (Peptic Ulcer)

****

Open sores that develop on the inside lining of your esophagus, stomach and the upper portion of your small intestine.

A stomach ulcer is a break in the tissue lining the stomach. About 60% of peptic ulcers are caused by the infection Helicobacter Pylori.

Symptoms of a Stomach Ulcer

- Abdominal pain just below the rib cage;
- Indigestion;
- Nausea and Vomiting;
- Loss of Appetite and/or Weight Loss;
- Blood in the vomit or bowels; or
- Symptoms of Anemia, such as light-headedness.

Causes of Stomach Ulcers

- An infection with Helicobacter Pylori;
- Long term use of NSAID's;
- Zollinger-Ellison Syndrome – Rare disease that makes the body produce excess stomach acid.

Factors that put people at greater risk of Stomach Ulcers

- Smoking;
- Frequent use of steroids;
- Hypercalcemia;
- Family history of stomach ulcers;
- Being over 50 years of age;
- Excessive consumption of alcohol.

How MSM can help Stomach Ulcers

An increase in MSM can stabilize your pH level, therefore helping to normalize stomach function and help prevent an overproduction of stomach acids. This will obviously help alleviate heartburn and stomach ulcers.

Recommended form and dosage of MSM for Stomach Ulcers

As with many other conditions the dosage will depend on your individual requirements. Start off with 1g per day and increase the dose until you start to notice improvements in your symptoms.

****

SECTION 3 – ADDITIONAL INFORMATION

****

Chapter #31 – Pets

****

So, MSM benefits humans in a multitude of ways (as discussed) but you would be interested to know that it is also extremely beneficial to your pets.

Is Your Dog Getting Enough MSM?

Unfortunately, even if your dog is consuming a raw, whole food diet may still not be getting enough MSM in their diet.

Nutritional Sources of MSM for your pet

If you are wanting to give your pet as much MSM as you possibly can with nutritional sources then try including as many of the following foods as possible to their meals:

- Bones;
- Raw Meat;
- Trachea;
- Connective Tissue.

Symptoms of Sulfur Deficiencies in Dogs

- Dull Fur;
- Skin Problems;
- Poor GI health;
- Lowered immunity;
- Joint Pain; and
- Arthritis.

Main Uses of MSM in Dogs

- Joint and Connective Tissue Support;
- Pain relief for arthritis, hip dysplasia and joint problems;
- Maintenance of healthy skin and hair;
- Relief of allergy symptoms.

Toxicity of MSM for Dogs

MSM has been used for years to treat joint disorders in pets.

71

Chapter #32 – Recipes

****

I thought it was only fitting to include some MSM recipes that you can make yourself all from the comfort of your own home. If you are requiring the ingredients you can gain access to them by doing any of the following:

Herbal Shampoo for Healthy Hair with MSM

I would like to recognize the website http://www.natural-homeremedies-for-life.com/homemade-shamp oo.html for some amazing homemade shampoo recipes with some awesome herbs.

Ingredients

2 Cups	Distilled Water
0.5 cup	Liquid Olive Oil/Castile Soap
10 drops	Rosemary Oil
10 drops	Lavender Oil
10 drops	Geranium Oil
2000mg	MSM

Methods

1. Boil the distilled water and in the meantime mix all the herbs in a small container.

2. Add 3 Tablespoons of the mixed herbs into the boiling water and stir very gently.

3. Take the pot off the heat source and let it sit for 35 minutes.

4. Let it cool for 30 minutes and then add the MSM.

5. Leave it for about 40 minutes so the MSM can melt.

6. Strain the mixture.

7. Pour ¼ cup of the liquid into a plastic bottle and add the liquid soap.

Pain Relief Cream with MSM

Ingredients

100mls	Base Cream
15g	Pure MSM Powder
10 drops	Lavender Essential Oil
10 drops	Peppermint Essential Oil
10 drops	Rosemary Essential Oil
10 drops	Thyme Essential Oil

Methods

1. Put 100mls of Base Cream into a bowl;

2. Place the MSM into a cup;

3. Add 2 tablespoons boiling water.

4. Cover the cup and place it in the microwave for 10 seconds. Check that the flakes are completely dissolved.

5. When fully dissolved, slowly add it to the cream and stir thoroughly.

6. Add the essential oils to the cream and mix completely.

Sinusitis Solution

Ingredients

1	Mini Spray Bottle
1 tsp	Pure MSM Powder (equiv 4g)
1 oz	Pure Filtered Water

Methods

Mix the Powder and Water together in the dropper or spray bottle and put a couple of drops or 3-4 sprays of this liquid into each nostril several times per day. Continue to do this until the sinusitis settles down. If you are prone to it and it is allergy season it may be worthwhile doing it even when you do not have sinusitis so as to try to ward it off.

Note: You may find that there is a little burning in the nostrils to start with but don't be alarmed. That will generally settle down within a few days, so persevere with it.

MSM Eye Drops or Eye Wash

Ingredients

Isotonic saline solution, found at any drug store
MSM Pure Powder Flakes (not the fine powder)
One dropper bottle

Methods

1. Heat 10 tbsp of saline solution in a small glass jar for a few minute

2. Add 1 tsp of MSM flakes and stir until it dissolves.

3. To use it as a wash you can use an eye wash cup and rinse the eyes with this solution.

4. To use it as an eye drop you can get a dropper bottle, put the mixture into it and then use 3-4 drops at a time.

5. *Please note this can cause your eye to sting when you first start using it so take it slowly.*

MSM Gel

Ingredients

100mls	Aloe Vera Gel
15g	MSM Pure Powder Flakes

Methods

1. Put 100mls of pure Aloe Vera Gel into a container or mixing bowl.

2. Add 15g of MSM (3 rounded tsp of crystal flakes) or more depending on how much Aloe Vera you are using.

3. Mix together.

4. To use it as a wash you can use an eye wash cup and rinse the eyes with this solution. To use as an eye drop you can get a dropper bottle, put the mixture into it and then use 3-4 drops at a time, especially when you have dry eyes. Please note this can cause your eye to sting when you first start using it so just persevere.

Conclusion

****

So, firstly I want to thank you for reading through to the end of the book. I am hoping by now that you are convinced how beneficial MSM can be for treating a multitude of conditions.

If you are suffering from any of the conditions listed or you find yourself dealing with extreme pain, then it may be worthwhile giving msm a go.

I consider MSM to be a supplement that everybody should have in their medicine cabinet, because if nothing else, it will certainly make you feel great.

3 Places You Can Get Magnesium...

Option #1 - Worldwide

No matter where you are, a good option for finding some suitable magnesium is finding a local health food store and seeing what magnesium they have on offer. Remember to take my book with you if possible so you can see what the best types of magnesium are for you.

Option #2 - Most countries (some only available in US) - Amazon via my store

I have sourced out some magnesium products that I believe are of great quality. If you would like to check this out, you can go to http://www.asknaturopathjen.com/store

Option #3 - Australia Only

If you live in Australia, you are able to contact me via email at jen@asknaturopathjen.com and let me know what you are requiring. I have suppliers where I can get some good quality supplements and I can have them shipped to you anywhere in Australia.

Free Inner Circle

Also, please don't forget to go to http://www.asknaturopathjen.com/innercircle and sign up for our mailing list. This will entitle you to free ebooks and/or courses as they come out, additional subscriber only articles and much more...

Testimonials

So, what are you waiting for? Get yourself some msm and see how great you can feel. Once you have tried it please email me at jen@asknaturopathjen.com and give me a testimonial on how MSM has helped you. This would be awesome!!!

Once again, thanks very much for reading my book. If you would like to check out the references associated with this book, please see below. I have spent a lot of time and effort researching all the information I have given, and I hope it has given you some insight into the amazing wonders of "MSM".

****

SECTION 4 – REFERENCES

****

Scientific References

****

1. Magnuson et al, 2006, Food and Chemical Toxicology, "Oral Developmental Toxicity Study of Methylsulfonylmethane (as OptiMSM®) in Rats."

2. Takiyama K et al, 2010, Oyo Yakuri Pharmacometrics, "Single and 13 – Week Repeated Oral Dose Toxicity of Methylsulfonylmethane in Mice".

3. Barrager E et al, The Journal of Alternative and Complementary Medicine, 2004, "A Multi-Centered, Open Label Trial on the safety and efficacy of Methylsulfonylmethane in the Treatment of Seasonal Allergic Rhinitis".

4. DiSilvestro R et al, 2008, FASEB, "Methylsulfonylmethane (MSM) Intake in Mice Produces Elevated Liver Glutathione and Partially Protects Against Carbon Tetrachloride-Induced Liver Injury".

5. Nakhostin-Roohi B, Iranian Journal of Pharmaceutical Research, 2013, "Effect of Single Dose administration of methylsulfonylmethane on oxidative stress following acute exhaustive exercise".

6. Kalman DS et al, Journal of International Society of Sports Nutrition, "Influence of methylsulfonylmethane on markers of exercise recovery and performance in healthy men: a pilot study".

7. Morton JI, Proceedings of the Society for Experimental Biology and Medicine, 1984, "Effects of oral dimethyl sulfoxide and dimethyl sulfone on murine autoimmune lymphoproliferative disease".

8. Kim JH et al, World Journal of Hepatology, 2014, "Methylsulfonylmethane suppresses hepatic tumor development through activation of apoptosis".

9. Lim EJ et al, PLoS One, 2012, "Methylsulfonylmethane suppresses breast cancer growth by down-regulating STAT3 and STAT5b pathways".

10. Caron JM et al, 2010, PLoS One, "Methyl sulfone induces loss of metastatic properties and re-emergence of normal phenotypes in a metastatic cloudman S-91 (M3) murine melanoma cell line".

11. Bohlooli S et al, Iranian Journal of Basic Medical Sciences, 2013, "Effect of methylsulfonylmethane pre-treatment on acetaminophen induced hepatotoxicity in rats".

12. Stanley Jacob et al, 1999, "The Miracle of MSM: The Natural Solution for Pain".

13. Ronald M Lawrence, MSM and Hair/Nail Health.

14. Amirshahrokhi K et al, Inflammation, 2013, "Effect of methylsulfonylmethane on paraquat induced acute lung and liver injury in mice."

15. Kamel, R et al, Archives of Pharmacal Research, 2013, "Hepatoprotective effect of methylsulfonylmethane against carbon tetrachloride-induced acute liver injury in rats".

16. Kim LS et al, Osteoarthritis Cartilage, 2006, "Efficacy of Methylsulfonylmethane (MSM) in Osteoarthritis pain of the knee: a pilot clinical trial.

17. Usha PR et al, Clinical Drug Investigation, 2004, "Randomised, Double Blind, Parallel, Placebo Controlled study of oral glucosamine, methylsulfonylmethane and their combination in osteoarthritis".

18. Lawrence RM, International Journal of Anti-Ageing Medicine, 1998, "Methylsulfonylmethane (M.S.M.) a double-blind study of use in degenerative arthritis".

19. Jacob S, "Pharmacologic Management of Snoring".

Website References

****

http://theshawnstevensonmodel.com/7-benefits-of-msm-the-mira cle-supplement/

http://www.msmguide.com/jointpain/improvejointhealth/

http://all-natural.com/msm.html

http://healthyeating.sfgate.com/major-sources-dietary-sulfur-4924. html

http://www.cancertutor.com/msm-article/

http://www.msmguide.com/facts/safety/

http://some-like-it-raw.com/2012/02/10/super-food-msm/

http://healthyeating.sfgate.com/major-sources-dietary-sulfur-4924. html

http://www.msmguide.com/facts/faq/

http://www.msmguide.com/facts/faq/

http://www.natural-health-and-healing-4u.com/msm-powder.html

http://www.naturodoc.com/library/medsmats/msm/MSM_backg round.htm

http://altmedsales.com/index.php?target=pages&page_id=MSM_ eyes

http://ezinearticles.com/?Improve-Your-Eye-Health-With-Natural -Remedies&id=914461

http://www.msm-info.com/

http://livingclean.com/msm-knowledge-base/msm-and-your-diges tive-health/

http://wellnessmama.com/5888/how-to-make-bone-broth/

http://www.nutritionexpress.com/showarticle.aspx?id=830

http://www.yearstoyourhealth.com/natural_calm/natural_vitality_info/msm.html

https://answers.yahoo.com/question/index?qid=20070702184959AAfQa7h

http://www.webmd.com/digestive-disorders/digestive-diseases-live r-failure

http://www.immunehealthscience.com/how-to-raise-glutathione.ht ml

http://aminoacidstudies.org/l-glutathione/

http://www.naturodoc.com/sulfurstudy.htm

http://www.gelout.com/pages/Athletic-Performance.html

http://www.askdrmaxwell.com/2013/06/autoimmune-disease-glutathione-n-acetyl-cysteine/

http://www.healingdaily.com/oral-chelation/MSM-for-detoxification.htm

http://www.flexquarters.com/getmsm/msm.htm

http://www.mindbodyhealth.com/RoexMSM.htm

http://en.wikipedia.org/wiki/Gastroesophageal_reflux_disease

http://www.totalhealthmagazine.com/articles/vitamins-and-supplements/what-is-msm.html

http://www.sleepeducation.com/essentials-in-sleep/snoring/cause s-and-symptoms

http://health.howstuffworks.com/wellness/natural-medicine/alternative/msm3.htm

http://www.natural-dog-health-remedies.com/msm-for-dogs.html

http://bestvitaminforhairgrowth.net/msm-for-hair-growth/

http://scdlifestyle.com/2010/03/the-scd-diet-and-leaky-gut-syndro me/

http://www.dazer.com/home/msm

http://www.mayoclinic.org/diseases-conditions/osteoarthritis/basi cs/causes/con-20014749

http://www.msmguide.com/jointpain/jointpainrelief/

http://www.arthritis-msm-supplements.com/Blog/?p=178

http://www.healthline.com/health/stomach-ulcer#Diagnosis4

http://www.medicalnewstoday.com/info/diabetes/

http://www.nwhealthsolutions.com/diabetes.htm

http://www.dogsnaturallymagazine.com/msm-raw-fed-dogs/